MANAGING

DIABETES

By

Jason Schnitzel

TABLE OF CONTENTS

INTRODUCTION

Diabetes can be difficult to live with, but with the correct information and resources, you can properly manage your health and maintain a happy, rewarding life.

This article attempts to offer thorough guidance on

controlling diabetes, from comprehending the fundamentals to creating a customised treatment strategy. This book will empower you to take charge of your health and well-being, regardless of how long you've had diabetes.

Comprehending Diabetes

Diabetes is a long-time period infection that affects

the body's cappotential to utilise meals as fuel. Most of the food you eat is normally converted by your body into sugar, or glucose, which is then released into your bloodstream.

Your pancreas releases insulin in reaction to an growth in blood sugar. Insulin functions as a key to allow blood sugar to enter your body's cells and be used as an energy source. When you have diabetes, your body is either unable to use the insulin it produces effectively or is unable to produce enough of it.

Too a good deal blood sugar stays for your circulate while there's inadequate insulin or while cells end reacting to insulin.

Serious health issues like renal disease, heart disease, and vision loss may result from this over time.

Diabetes: What is it?

Diabetes is a metabolic disease marked by elevated blood glucose (sugar) levels. It happens when the body either produces insufficient insulin, the hormone that controls blood sugar, or when the cells in the body do not react to insulin as they should. Diabetes comes in three different forms: gestational type 1, type 2, and type 1.

An autoimmune disease in which the body targets and kills the pancreatic beta cells that produce insulin.

Causes: Environmental and genetic variables; frequently

identified during childhood or adolescence.

Management: Needs lifetime insulin medication in addition to close observation of blood sugar levels, nutrition, and physical activity.

Diabetes Type 2

A disorder in which the pancreas fails to produce enough insulin or in which the body develops resistance to insulin.

Causes: More common in adults but increasingly observed in younger people; frequently associated with lifestyle choices, obesity, and hereditary factors.

Management: Oral medicines, insulin therapy,

dietary and exercise modifications, and other lifestyle strategies are used.

Diabetes during pregnancy

This type of diabetes typically goes away after giving delivery and arises during pregnancy.

Causes: Pregnancy-related hormonal changes can increase cellular resistance to insulin.

Management: Controlled by food, exercise, and occasionally insulin; vital to keep an eye on since it may have an impact on the health of the mother and child.

Signs and Prognosis Common Diabetes Symptoms:
• recurring urination

heightened hunger and thirst

• Unexpected weight reduction

• Weary

• hazy vision

• recurrent infections or slow-healing wounds

Conclusion:

Abstinence Test for Blood Sugar: After an overnight fast, blood glucose is measured. When the result is 126 mg/dL or over, diabetes is suspected.

The A1C test shows the average blood sugar levels over the previous two to three months. When the A1C is 6.5% or more, diabetes is suspected.

Blood glucose is measured both before and after consuming a sweet beverage using the oral glucose tolerance test (OGTT). After two hours, levels 200 mg/dL or above suggest diabetes.

A blood sample drawn at random for a blood sugar test. Diabetes is suggested by a result of 200 mg/dL or greater, particularly if symptoms are present.

The Value of Prompt Identification and Treatment

To avoid or postpone problems, diabetes must be identified early and managed well.

Cardiovascular illness, nerve damage (neuropathy), kidney

damage (nephropathy), eye damage (retinopathy), and foot issues are some of the difficulties that might impact different body parts.

Important Management Techniques:
Regular Monitoring:
Monitoring blood sugar levels to help guide decisions regarding medicine, nutrition, and activity.

Eating Healthily: Consuming a balanced diet that aids with blood sugar regulation.

Physical Activity: Maintaining a healthy weight and enhancing insulin sensitivity can be achieved by frequent physical activity.

Medication adherence refers to taking prescription drugs as instructed by medical professionals.

Education and Support: Keeping up with diabetes-related information and asking family, friends, and medical professionals for assistance.

CHAPTER 1:

TAKING CHARGE OF YOUR HEALTH

When managing diabetes, it's important to take control of your health by developing a thorough care plan, collaborating closely with medical providers, establishing reasonable objectives, and scheduling routine check-ups and monitoring.

The crucial actions in this chapter will assist you in controlling your diabetes and enhancing your general health.

Creating a Care Plan for Diabetes

A diabetes care plan is a customized road map created to assist you in successfully managing your disease. It consists of modifications to lifestyle, medicine, routines for monitoring, and approaches to avoid complications. collaborating with your medical group.

Your major source of help when managing your diabetes is your healthcare team. Usually, it consists of: Your diabetes care is coordinated by your primary care physician (PCP).

Endocrinologist: Focuses on hormone imbalances and diabetes.

Nutritionists and dietitians: Offer advice on meal preparation and healthful eating.
A diabetes educator provides information and assistance with managing diabetes.

Pharmacist: Provides guidance and assistance with drug management.

Optometrists and ophthalmologists: Keep an eye on things to avoid diabetic retinopathy.

Podiatrist: Offers foot treatment to avoid problems.

Important Actions for Creating a Care Plan:
First Assessment: Assess your present health condition, including blood pressure, cholesterol, blood sugar, A1C, and other pertinent health markers, in collaboration with your healthcare team.

Establishing Objectives:
Establish realistic short-term and long-term goals for blood sugar control, weight management, physical exercise, and other elements of diabetes treatment.

Schedule of Monitoring:
Establish a routine for routine blood pressure checks, A1C tests, blood

sugar checks, and other required monitoring.

Medication Management: Make a schedule for taking insulin, prescription drugs, over-the-counter medications, and any additional therapies.

Lifestyle Modifications: Determine the precise lifestyle modifications you must implement, such as food modifications, heightened physical activity, and stress reduction methods.

Having Reasonable Objectives

Achievable goals are essential for managing diabetes effectively. Objectives have to be time-bound, relevant, quantifiable, attainable, and specific (SMART).

Instances of Practical Objectives:

Blood Sugar Control: As directed by your healthcare practitioner, try to keep your blood glucose levels within the target range.

A1C Levels: Try to bring your A1C down to less than 7%, or as directed by your physician.

Diet and Nutrition: Make an effort to eat fewer processed and sugar-filled foods and increase your intake of lean meats, vegetables, and whole grains.

Physical Activity: Try to get in at least 150 minutes a week of moderate-to-intense activity, such swimming, cycling, or walking.

Weight management: If you are overweight, make it a goal to reduce 5–10% of your body weight. Even a small amount of weight lost can have a big impact on blood sugar regulation.

Stress Reduction: Make time each day for stress-relieving practices like yoga, meditation, or deep breathing techniques.

Frequent observation and evaluation

Effective management of your diabetes requires routinely assessing your health. This include taking your own blood pressure every day, getting tested for A1C on a regular basis, and visiting your doctor on a regular basis.

Tracking Blood Sugar Levels:

Self-Monitoring: As directed by your healthcare practitioner, monitor your blood sugar levels with a blood glucose meter. To spot trends and modify your care plan as needed, keep a record of your readings.

Continuous glucose monitoring (CGM): If your doctor advises it, think about utilizing a CGM device. With the support of real-time glucose readings and trends from CGMs, you may make better educated choices regarding your diet, exercise routine, and prescription drugs.

Frequent Examinations:

A1C Tests: If necessary, get your A1C levels checked more frequently than twice a year. An average blood sugar level for the previous two to three months is provided by the A1C test.

Blood pressure and cholesterol: To lower your chance of developing cardiovascular problems, check your blood pressure and cholesterol levels on a regular basis.

Eye Exams: To look for indications of diabetic retinopathy, get a thorough eye checkup at least once a year.

Foot Exams: Check your feet every day for sores, blisters, and cuts. To avoid issues, schedule routine foot checkups with a podiatrist.

Through self-management and close collaboration with your healthcare team, you may create a diabetic care plan that works, establish attainable goals, and guarantee routine testing and examinations. These actions are crucial for both controlling your diabetes and preserving your general health and wellbeing.

CHAPTER 2
NUTRITION AND DIET

Diet has a critical role in the control of diabetes.

Knowing how different foods affect your blood sugar levels and general health can help you make decisions that support your diabetes management approach.

This chapter provides in-depth guidance on creating balanced meal plans, understanding macronutrients, and implementing healthy eating habits.

The Role of Nutrition in Diabetes Management

Eating right is essential for preventing issues, boosting general health, and keeping blood sugar levels within your target range. An essential part of diabetes diet is understanding the impacts of fats, proteins, and carbohydrates and making informed meal choices.

An Awareness of Fats, Carbohydrates, and Proteins

Function: Carbohydrates are the body's primary energy source. Their effects are directly felt on blood sugar levels.

Types: Simple carbohydrates (sugars) and complicated carbohydrates (starches and fibers).

Impact on Blood Sugar Levels: Simple carbohydrates cause blood sugar to rise quickly, while complex carbohydrates release glucose more gradually over time.

Proteins:
Function: Proteins are essential for the growth and repair of tissues and have minimal effect on blood sugar levels.

Among the sources include lean meats, poultry, fish, eggs, dairy products, legumes, nuts, and seeds.

Impact on Blood Sugar: Proteins can keep blood sugar levels steady and extend sensations of fullness.

Lipids:

Function: Fats are a concentrated source of energy and are necessary for the absorption of fat-soluble vitamins. Saturated fats, monounsaturated and polyunsaturated unsaturated fats, and trans fats are among the varieties.

Effect on Blood Sugar:
Despite the fact that fats
don't directly affect blood
sugar levels, using them in
moderation is still important
for heart health.

**Creating a Sophisticated
Meal Plan**
A balanced meal plan
includes foods from all the
food groups, ensuring you
get the nutrients you need

while keeping your blood sugar levels under control.

How to Create a Meal Plan with Good Balance:

Eat a Variety of Foods: Take in fruits, vegetables, whole grains, lean meats, and healthy fats.

Control of Portion: Consider portion sizes to avoid overindulging and maintain stable blood sugar levels.

Calculating Carbohydrates: Keep track of how many carbohydrates you consume at each meal and snack.

Consistency: Try to eat meals and snacks at the same time each day to help control blood sugar levels.

Drinking plenty of water
Avoid sugar-filled drinks
and drink lots of water.

The Glycemic Index: Crucial Details

The glycemic index (GI) indicates how quickly a carbohydrate-rich meal raises blood sugar levels.

High GI foods cause rapid spikes in blood sugar levels,

while low GI foods cause a slower, more gradual rise.

Foods low in glycerol: vegetables (broccoli, spinach, tomatoes) that aren't starchy

Whole grains: brown rice, quinoa, and oats
Legumes (beans, lentils)
a few fruits, including apples, berries, and pears

High GI Foods:
White bread and refined grains, sweet snacks and treats
Cornflakes and sweet potatoes
Increasing the quantity of low-GI foods in your diet will help maintain stable blood sugar levels.

Particular Diets: Low-Carb, Mediterranean, and Other Diets

Reducing carbohydrate intake to improve blood sugar management is the main point.

Foods to Include: Lean proteins, non-starchy vegetables, and healthy fats.

Benefits: May lead to reduced weight and better blood sugar regulation.

**The Diet of the
Mediterranean
Focus:** Gives nuts, olive oil,
fruits, vegetables, whole
grains, and legumes a lot of
attention.

Foods to Incorporate:
Fish, poultry, lentils, and

dairy products in moderation.

Benefits: Promotes heart health and stable blood sugar levels.

Alternative Diets: Consult a nutritionist about alternative nutritional approaches that may be more suitable for your specific circumstances, such as plant-based diets or the DASH diet.

Organising and Setting Up Meals

With the right meal planning and preparation, eating healthily may be simpler and more reliable.

Methods for Preparing Healthy Foods

Grilling, steaming, and baking reduce the need for extra fat.

Using Herbs and Spices: Leave off the sugar and salt to enhance flavour.

Batch cooking: Make meals ahead of time to ensure you have healthful selections available and to save time.

Analyzing Nutrition Labels
Knowing what food labels
mean might help you make
informed selections.

Serving Dimensions:
Check the serving size to
determine the specific
amount of carbohydrates
and other nutrients.
include fibre, sugars, and
starches among its total

carbs. Pay interest to the quantity of delivered sugars.

Fats and Sodium: Limit the amount of sodium, trans fats, and saturated fats you consume.

Social Events and Outside Dining

While going to social gatherings and eating out

can be challenging, you can make healthy choices if you prepare ahead of time: Look over menus ahead of time and choose restaurants that have a good assortment of healthier options.

Control Portion Sizes: Consider bringing some food home with you or splitting a meal.

Organize your plate such that it has a range of nutritious vegetables, cereals, and proteins.

Converse with one another: Never be scared to ask for modifications to your dish, such as dressing on the side or grilled instead of fried.

CHAPTER 3
PHYSICAL ACTIVITY

Exercise is one of the most crucial parts of diabetic management. Regular exercise improves overall health, reduces blood sugar, and enhances quality of life. This chapter explores the importance of physical activity, how it affects blood sugar levels, types of exercise, creating a personalized training plan, and methods for staying motivated and safe.

The Benefits of Exercise
Exercise is beneficial for everyone, but those with diabetes especially need to be aware of this. Regular exercise has a number of advantages, including: Improved Blood Sugar Control: By helping the muscles use glucose as

fuel, exercise decreases blood sugar levels. Weight management: Exercise helps to maintain a healthy weight by lowering insulin resistance.

Cardiovascular Health: Regular exercise strengthens the heart and improves circulation.

Mental Health: Physical activity reduces tension, anxiety, and symptoms of depression.

Increased Energy: Engaging in physical activity reduces fatigue and increases overall energy levels.

How Exercise Affects Blood Sugar

Physical activity affects blood sugar levels in a number of ways:

Exercise reduces blood sugar levels during and after exercise by improving cell utilisation of glucose and increasing insulin sensitivity. These benefits are felt immediately.

Consequences: Following physical activity, blood sugar levels may remain decreased for hours due to the increased sensitivity to insulin.

Preventing Highs and Lows: Regular exercise can help reduce blood sugar fluctuation overall and help prevent spikes in blood sugar after meals.

Nonetheless, it's important to be aware of the risk of hypoglycemia, or low blood sugar, before and after physical activity, especially for those on insulin or other diabetic medications. It is imperative to monitor blood sugar levels before, during, and after physical activity.

Types of Exercise:
Strength, Flexibility, and Aerobic
Including a variety of exercises in your program has multiple health benefits:

Cardiovascular Work:
Exercises that increase heart rate and breathing. Among them include jogging, cycling, swimming, dancing, and walking.

Benefits include increased enjoyment, burning calories, and better cardiovascular health.

Exercises designed to improve muscle strength and endurance are referred to as strengthening exercises.
Weightlifting, resistance band exercises, and bodyweight exercises

(squats, push-ups) are a few examples.

Benefits: Increases muscle mass, metabolism, and insulin sensitivity. Activities designed to improve flexibility, balance, and coordination are referred to as adaptation and equilibrium.

For example, stretching, yoga, and tai chi. Increased range of motion, a decreased risk of injury, and relaxation are some advantages.

Creating a Tailored Exercise Program

A personalised exercise plan should take into account your current level of fitness, general health, and your goals for controlling your diabetes. Here's how to create one:

Assess Your Current Fitness Level: Consider your current level of physical activity, any limitations, and any health concerns.

Make sure you consult your physician prior to starting a new exercise regimen.

Set logical goals:
Set SMART objectives, which stand for specific, measurable, achievable, relevant, and time-bound. For example: "Five days a week, I will walk for thirty minutes.

Choose Your Enjoyment Activities:
Select athletic pursuits that fit with your schedule and that you enjoy.

Include a variety of workouts in your schedule to keep it interesting and well-rounded.

Make a Schedule: Plan regular workouts, ideally at the same time each day, to help break the habit.

Aim for at least 150 minutes of moderate-intensity aerobic activity each week in addition to two to three strength training sessions per week.

Keeping Yourself Safe and Motivated While Exercising

Maintaining motivation and ensuring safety are crucial elements of a successful exercise program:

Sustaining Inspiration:
Decide on short-term goals:
Break down your long-term
goals into smaller, more
achievable criteria.

Track Development: Use
fitness programs or an
exercise log to monitor your
progress.

**Locate a Training
Companion:** Exercise with
a friend or in a club can

boost accountability and enjoyment.

Give a Treat to Yourself: Give yourself a non-food reward for your achievements, such as new exercise gear or a calming hobby.

Maintaining Everyone's Safety:

Observe your blood sugar: Check your blood sugar before, during, and after physical exercise, as well as whenever you start a new activity.

Preserve Hydration: Drink plenty of water prior to, during, and following physical activity.

Put on the Proper Footwear: Wear supportive, comfy shoes to prevent foot injury.

Warm-Up and Cool-Down: Perform warm-up exercises before your workout and cool-down stretches afterward to help prevent injury.

Observe Your Body: While working out, become aware

of how your body is feeling.
If you get dizziness,
shortness of breath, or
chest pain, stop and seek
medical attention.

CHAPTER 3
PHYSICAL ACTIVITY

One of the most important aspects of diabetic care is physical activity. Frequent exercise raises quality of life, lowers blood sugar, and improves general health.

This chapter delves into the significance of physical activity, its impact on blood sugar levels, various forms of exercise, designing a customized workout regimen, and strategies for maintaining motivation and safety.

The Value of Physical Activity

Everyone benefits from exercise, but those who have diabetes should take particular note of this. Frequent exercise has several benefits, such as:

Better Blood Sugar Control:
Exercise lowers blood sugar levels by assisting the muscles in using glucose as fuel.

Weight management:
Exercise lowers insulin resistance and aids in maintaining a healthy weight.

Cardiovascular Health: Frequent exercise enhances circulation and fortifies the heart.

Mental Health: Exercise helps lower stress, anxiety, and depressive symptoms.

Enhanced Energy: Physical activity elevates one's general energy levels and mitigates weariness.

How Blood Sugar Is Affected by Exercise

There are various ways that physical activity influences

blood sugar levels:

Exercise has immediate effects via raising insulin sensitivity, which improves cell use of glucose and lowers blood sugar levels both during and after exercise.

Repercussions:
Because of the enhanced sensitivity to insulin, blood sugar levels may stay lowered for hours following physical activity.

Preventing Highs and Lows:
Engaging in regular physical activity will help lower overall blood sugar variability and avoid blood sugar rises following meals.

But, it's crucial to be mindful of the possibility of hypoglycemia (low blood sugar) both before and after physical activity, particularly for people on insulin or other diabetic treatments.

It's critical to check blood sugar levels prior to, during, and following exercise.
Exercise Types: Aerobic, Strength, and Flexibility

Including a range of workouts in your program offers several health

Advantages:
Benefits include calorie burning, improved happiness, and improved cardiovascular health.

Strength training:
Exercises designed to increase muscle endurance and strength.

Examples include bodyweight exercises (squats, push-ups), resistance band exercises, and weightlifting.

Benefits: Boosts insulin sensitivity, increases muscle mass, and increases metabolism. Activities that enhance coordination, balance, and flexibility are referred to as flexibility and balance activities.

For instance, tai chi, yoga, and stretching.
Benefits include increased range of motion, less chance of injury, and relaxation.

Formulating a Customised Workout Program
Your fitness level, overall health, and your objectives

for managing your diabetes should all be reflected in a customized workout program.

This is how to make one:
Determine Your Present State of Fitness
Take into account your degree of physical activity right now, as well as any restrictions or medical issues.

Be positive to talk together along with your physician earlier than starting a brand new health program.

For instance: "I will walk for 30 minutes, five days a week.

Select Pleasure-Seeking Activities

Choose physical activities that you enjoy and that work with your schedule.

To maintain the fun and balance of your regimen, incorporate a variety of workouts.

Establish a Timetable
To create a habit, schedule frequent workouts, ideally at the same time every day.

Aim for two to three times a week of strength training exercises in addition to at least 150 minutes of moderate-intensity aerobic activity per week.

Maintaining Safety and Motivation During Exercise

Retaining motivation and guaranteeing security are essential components of an effective workout regimen:

Maintaining Motivation

Set Temporary Objectives: Divide your long-term objectives into more manageable benchmarks.

Track Your Progress: You can track your progress by using fitness apps or by keeping an activity log.

Find a Workout Partner: Joining a club or working

out with a friend can increase enjoyment and accountability.

Give Yourself a Treat: Reward yourself for your accomplishments with non-food items like new fitness equipment or a soothing pastime.

Taking Care of Safety Monitor Blood Sugar: Whenever you begin a new activity or before, during, or after physical activity, check your blood sugar levels.

Maintain Hydration: Before, during, and after exercise, sip lots of water. Wear Appropriate Footwear: To avoid foot injuries, select comfortable, supportive footwear.

Warm-Up and Cool-Down: To help prevent injuries,

use warm-up movements prior to your workout and cool-down stretches following it.

Pay Attention to Your Body: During exercising, pay attention to how your body feels. Stop and get medical help if you develop shortness of breath, dizziness, or chest pain.

CHAPTER 4

MONITORING AND MANAGING BLOOD SUGAR

Good blood sugar control and monitoring are essential for diabetes patients to preserve their health and avoid problems.

This chapter offers in-depth information on the significance of blood sugar monitoring, different monitoring techniques, comprehension of blood sugar levels, and blood sugar management tactics.

The Significance of Monitoring Blood Sugar

You can better understand how various factors, such as diet, exercise, medication, and stress, affect your blood sugar levels by regularly testing your blood sugar.

Critical information obtained from monitoring can assist you in:

Make Well-Informed Choices: Based on real-time data, modify your medicine, food, and level of physical activity.

Avoid Complications: Steer clear of hypoglycemia (low blood sugar) and hyperglycemia (high blood sugar), as these conditions can cause major health problems.

Monitor Development: Keep an eye on the effectiveness of your diabetes management strategy and make any required modifications.

Interact with Healthcare Professionals: Give your medical staff precise information so they can customise your course of therapy.

Techniques for Monitoring Blood Sugar
There are numerous ways to keep an eye on your blood sugar levels:

Using a blood glucose metre for self-monitoring of blood glucose (SMBG):

Steps: Clean your hands, set up the test strip and metre.

Using a lancet, prick your fingertip to extract a drop of blood.

After placing the blood drop on the test strip, watch for

the result to appear on the metre.

Frequency: Depending on your treatment plan, your healthcare professional will advise you on how frequently to test your blood sugar.

Using a CGM device for continuous glucose monitoring (CGM):

Parts: A receiver or smartphone app, a transmitter connected to the tiny sensor placed beneath the skin, and a receiver.

Function: Every few minutes, the sensor detects the amount of glucose in the interstitial fluid and transmits data to the receiver.

Benefits: Offers trends, alarms for high or low blood sugar, and real-time glucose measurements.

Knowing Your Blood Sugar Levels

Understanding how to interpret your blood sugar results is crucial for managing your diabetes effectively. The following are some essential ideas:

Goal Blood Sugar Levels
General Objectives (may change depending on personal objectives and health conditions):

Before meals, on a fast: 80–130 mg/dL
Less than 180 mg/dL postprandial (1-2 hours after meals) and 100–140 mg/dL at bedtime

Identifying Trends and Patterns

Every Day Variations: Observe how your blood sugar reacts to meals, exercise, and medications throughout the course of the day.

Weekly Patterns: Seek out reoccurring trends that can help you modify your diabetes care strategy.

Techniques for Controlling Blood Sugar

It takes a mix of medication management, lifestyle modifications, and routine monitoring to keep your blood sugar within your goal range. Here are a few successful tactics:

Nutrition and Dietary

Balanced Diet:

Counting carbs: Keep tabs on how many carbs you eat to prevent blood sugar rises.

Make healthy choices by emphasising whole grains, lean meats, omega-3 fatty acids, and an abundance of vegetables.

Low Glycemic Index Foods:
To avoid sharp spikes in blood sugar, choose for foods low on the GI scale.

Exercise
Frequent Workout:
activity Types: Include strength training, flexibility training, and aerobic activity.

Consistency: Try to get in at least 150 minutes a week of moderate-to-intense aerobic exercise. Medication Administration Compliance with Medication:

Insulin Therapy: Adhere to the schedule and dosage of your insulin as directed by your doctor.

Oral Medications: Follow your doctor's instructions when taking oral diabetic medications.

Modifying Drug Regimen: In Discussion with Medical Professionals: Consult your medical team to modify your medication regimen in light of your general health and blood sugar levels.

Stress Reduction
Taking Stress Off:

Techniques: Engage in relaxation exercises like yoga, meditation, or deep breathing.

Frequent rests: To prevent burnout and preserve mental health, take regular rests.

Keeping an eye on and modifying your plan
Frequent Check-Ins:

Regular Monitoring: As directed, check your blood sugar levels and modify your management strategy.

Professional Advice: Schedule routine check-ups with your physician so that you can go over your blood sugar records and make any required corrections.

CHAPTER 5

LIFESTYLE AND BEHAVIOURAL STRATEGIES

Living with diabetes means adopting regular behavioural and lifestyle adjustments that promote your general well-being in addition to taking medication as prescribed.

This chapter covers key techniques to support you in managing stress, incorporating good behaviors into your daily life, and adhering to your diabetes treatment plan.

Developing Healthful Routines

For diabetes to be effectively managed, it is essential to establish and maintain healthy habits.

The following techniques will assist you in creating and maintaining these habits:

Creating a Continual and Regular Daily Schedule:

Meals: To assist control blood sugar levels, eat meals and snacks at the same times every day.

Exercise: To make sure you stay active, set aside regular times for physical activity.

Frequent Observation: Blood Sugar Checks: Check your blood sugar levels daily at the same times to see trends and make any required corrections.

Having Reasonable Objectives

SMART Objectives:

Particular: Specify exactly what you want to achieve (for example, "I will walk for 30 minutes after dinner five days a week").

Measurable: Monitor your development by keeping a journal of your workouts or using a fitness tracker.

Attainable: Establish goals that are appropriate for your lifestyle and current level of fitness.

Relevant: Make sure your objectives and diabetes control strategy are in line.

Time-bound: Establish due dates (e.g., "I will achieve this by the end of the month") to help you reach your objectives.

Controlling Tension

Stress has a major effect on blood sugar levels and general health. Using practical stress-reduction strategies is essential to keeping diabetes under control.

Techniques for Relaxation:

Deep Breathing: To relax your body and mind, engage in deep breathing exercises.

Meditation: To lower stress, practice mindfulness or meditation.

Yoga: Include yoga in your regimen to help you unwind

both physically and mentally.

Exercise: Getting regular exercise lowers stress and elevates mood.

Nature Walks: Take some time to unwind and refresh yourself in the great outdoors.

Time management Task Prioritization:

Crucial versus urgent: Keep your attention on the essentials and resist the temptation to multitask on less important but urgent duties.

Divide Work into Steps: Break up more difficult jobs into smaller, more doable steps to lower stress and boost output.

Improving the Quality of Your Sleep

Good diabetes management and general health depend on getting enough sleep. Stress and blood sugar levels can both be impacted by little sleep.

Practices for Sleep Hygiene Consistent Sleep Schedule:

Regular Bedtime: Even on the weekends, go to bed

and wake up at the same hours every day.

Sleep Environment: Keep your bedroom quiet, dark, and cold to create a good sleeping environment.

Pre-nighttime routine:

Wind down: Create a calming bedtime ritual, like reading a book or having a warm bath.

Limit Screen Time: To enhance the quality of your sleep, avoid using screens (TVs, phones, and tablets) at least an hour before bed.

Maintaining Contact and Assistance

Having social support is essential for both controlling diabetes and keeping a good mindset.

Creating a Support System with Friends and Family:

Communicate: Let your loved ones know about your diabetes control objectives and difficulties.

Involvement: Get your loved ones and friends involved in your hobbies, such meal planning and working out together.

Support Teams:
Join Conversations: Join an online or in-person diabetes support group to meet people going through similar struggles.

Share Experiences: Group members should trade advice, anecdotes, and words of support.

Maintaining Knowledge and Education

Keeping up to date on the most recent findings, methods, and therapies for diabetes control is made easier with ongoing education.

Healthcare Providers and Educational Resources:

Make Regular Appointments:
To be informed about your health condition and management plan, schedule routine check-ups with your healthcare provider.

Pose inquiries: Never be afraid to clarify things and ask questions regarding your health and course of therapy.

Teaching Resources:

Books and Articles: To increase your understanding of diabetes management, read books and articles.

Online Courses: Attend webinars or online courses that respectable diabetes organisations are offering.

Taking Care of Your Emotional Health

Having diabetes can be emotionally taxing. It's critical to look after and maintain your mental well-being.

Strategies for Emotional Health

Acknowledge Your Feelings:

Acknowledge Emotions: Whether they are feelings of worry, despair, or frustration, acknowledge and accept them.

Express Emotions: Share your thoughts and feelings with a therapist, family member, or trusted friend.

Positivity in Thought: Put Progress First: Honour your accomplishments, no matter how modest, and concentrate on the strides you've achieved.

Remain Upbeat: Practise self-talk and gratitude to help you develop a happy outlook.
Including Behavioral and Lifestyle Changes

To properly manage diabetes, behavioural and

lifestyle measures must be combined.

Customised Action Plan Combining Techniques:

Holistic Approach: Incorporate into your everyday life good habits, stress reduction, restful sleep, social support, ongoing education, and emotional wellness.

Track Development:
Evaluate your progress on a regular basis and revise your plan as necessary. Modify and Align:

Flexibility: Adjust your tactics in response to your changing demands and situations. Be adaptable.

Seek Support: When in need, ask family, friends, and medical professionals for assistance.

You may improve the way your diabetes is managed, your general health, and your quality of life are maintained by putting these lifestyle and behavioral measures into practice.

To reach your objectives, stick to your plan, ask for help when you need it, and make changes as you go.

CHAPTER 6

COMPLICATIONS AND SPECIAL CONSIDERATION

Living with diabetes means adopting regular behavioural and lifestyle adjustments that promote your general well-being in addition to taking medication as prescribed.

This chapter covers key techniques to support you in managing stress, incorporating good behaviors into your daily life, and adhering to your diabetes treatment plan.

Developing Healthful Routines

For diabetes to be effectively managed, it is essential to establish and maintain healthy habits.

The following techniques will assist you in creating and maintaining these habits:

Creating a Continual and Regular Daily Schedule:

Meals: To assist control blood sugar levels, eat meals and snacks at the same times every day.

Exercise: To make sure you stay active, set aside regular times for physical activity.

Frequent Observation:

Blood Sugar Checks: Check your blood sugar levels daily at the same times to see trends and make any required corrections.

Particular: Specify exactly what you want to achieve (for example, "I will walk for 30 minutes after dinner five days a week").

Measurable: Monitor your development by keeping a journal of your workouts or using a fitness tracker.

Attainable: Establish goals that are appropriate for your lifestyle and current level of fitness.

Relevant: Make sure your objectives and diabetes control strategy are in line.

Time-bound: Establish due dates (e.g., "I will achieve this by the end of the month") to help you reach your objectives.
Controlling Tension

Stress has a major effect on blood sugar levels and general health. Using practical stress-reduction strategies is essential to keeping diabetes under control.

Techniques for Relaxation:
Deep Breathing: To relax your body and mind,

engage in deep breathing exercises.

Meditation: To lower stress, practice mindfulness or meditation.

Yoga: Include yoga in your regimen to help you unwind both physically and

Exercise: Getting regular exercise lowers stress and elevates mood..

Nature Walks: Take some time to unwind and refresh yourself in the great outdoors.

Time management Task Prioritization:

Crucial versus urgent: Keep your attention on the

essentials and resist the temptation to multitask on less important but urgent duties.

Divide Work into Steps: Break up more difficult jobs into smaller, more doable steps to lower stress and boost output.

Improving the Quality of Your Sleep

Good diabetes management and general health depend on getting enough sleep. Stress and blood sugar levels can both be impacted by little sleep.

Practices for Sleep Hygiene
Consistent Sleep Schedule:

Regular Bedtime: Even on the weekends, go to bed and wake up at the same hours every day.

Sleep Environment: Keep your bedroom quiet, dark, and cold to create a good sleeping environment. Pre-nighttime routine:

Wind down: Create a calming bedtime ritual, like

reading a book or having a warm bath.

Limit Screen Time: To enhance the quality of your sleep, avoid using screens (TVs, phones, and tablets) at least an hour before bed.

Maintaining Contact and Assistance

Having social support is essential for both controlling diabetes and keeping a good mindset.

Creating a Support System with Friends and Family:

Communicate: Let your loved ones know about your diabetes control objectives and difficulties.

Involvement: Get your loved ones and friends involved in your hobbies, such meal planning and working out together.

Support Teams:

Join Conversations: Join an online or in-person diabetes support group to meet people going through similar struggles.

Share Experiences: Group members should trade advice, anecdotes, and words of support.

Maintaining Knowledge and Education

Keeping up to date on the most recent findings, methods, and therapies for diabetes control is made easier with ongoing education.

Healthcare Providers and Educational Resources:

Make Regular Appointments: To be informed about your health condition and management plan, schedule routine check-ups with your healthcare provider.

Pose inquiries: Never be afraid to clarify things and ask questions regarding your health and course of therapy.

Teaching Resources:

Books and Articles: To increase your understanding of diabetes management, read books and articles.

Online Courses: Attend webinars or online courses that respectable diabetes organisations are offering.

Taking Care of Your Emotional Health

Having diabetes can be emotionally taxing. It's critical to look after and maintain your mental well-being.

Strategies for Emotional Health

Acknowledge Your Feelings:

Acknowledge Emotions:
Whether they are feelings of worry, despair, or frustration, acknowledge and accept them.

Express Emotions: Share your thoughts and feelings with a therapist, family member, or trusted friend. Positivity in Thought:

Put Progress First:
Honour your accomplishments, no matter how modest, and concentrate on the strides you've achieved.

Remain Upbeat: Practise self-talk and gratitude to help you develop a happy outlook.
Including Behavioral and Lifestyle Changes

To properly manage diabetes, behavioural and lifestyle measures must be combined.

Customised Action Plan Combining Techniques: Holistic Approach: Incorporate into your everyday life good habits, stress reduction, restful sleep, social support, ongoing education, and emotional wellness.

Track Development: Evaluate your progress on a regular basis and revise your plan as necessary.

Flexibility: Adjust your tactics in response to your changing demands and situations. Be adaptable.

Seek Support: When in need, ask family, friends,

and medical professionals for assistance.

You may improve the way your diabetes is managed, your general health, and your quality of life are maintained by putting these lifestyle and behavioural measures into practice. To reach your objectives, stick to your plan, ask for help when you need it, and make changes as you go.

CHAPTER 7
TECHNOLOGY AND INNOVATIONS

Technological developments have brought about a substantial transformation in the treatment of diabetes by providing new instruments and strategies for more efficient management. This chapter examines new developments in diabetes research, treatment approaches, and upcoming technology, emphasizing how these advancements can enhance the lives of those who have the disease.

New Technologies in the Management of Diabetes

As a result of ongoing technological advancements, diabetes can now be better monitored, managed, and treated.

The overall management of diseases as well as accuracy and convenience are the goals of these improvements.

Progress in Glucose Tracking

CGM, or continuous glucose monitoring:

Function: Using a sensor inserted beneath the skin, CGM devices deliver real-time glucose readings every few minutes.

Benefits: Reduces the risk of problems by providing users with notifications for high or low blood sugar levels, helping to recognize patterns, and providing ongoing insight into glucose trends.

Medtronic Guardian, FreeStyle Libre, and Dexcom are a few examples.

FGM, or flash glucose monitoring:

Function: Same as CGM, but to obtain a glucose reading, you must scan a sensor using a reader or smartphone.

Benefits: Offers comprehensive glucose data and is less invasive than conventional fingerstick testing. FreeStyle Libre is one example.

Insulin Delivery Systems and Pumps

Function: Insulin pumps replicate the pancreas' normal insulin release by continuously supplying insulin through a catheter inserted beneath the skin.

Benefits: include accurate insulin delivery, a reduction in the number of daily injections required, and the ability to modify dosage in response to glucose levels.

Tandem t:slim X2, Omnipod, and Medtronic

MiniMed are a few examples.

Automated Pancreatic Artificial Insulin Delivery Systems:

Function: Combines insulin pump and CGM technologies to automatically modify insulin dosage in response to blood glucose levels.

Benefits: By automating insulin adjustments, it improves glucose control and lessens the stress of managing diabetes. Tandem Control-IQ and Medtronic 670G are two examples.

Smartphone Applications and Web-Based Materials Apps for Diabetes Management:

Function: Use smartphone interfaces that are easy to use to monitor blood sugar levels, nutrition, exercise, and medicine.

Benefits: Offer data analysis, guidance, and reminders for improved diabetic care.
Glooko, Glucose Buddy, and mySugr are a few examples.

Telemedicine:

Function: Enables online messages, phone conversations, or video calls for remote consultations with medical professionals.

Benefits: include a decrease in the need for in-person visits, increased accessibility to medical advice, and continuous care.

Research on Diabetes in the Future Directions
The goals of diabetes care research are to create novel medications, enhance already-effective ones, and eventually discover a cure.

These are a few exciting areas of present and upcoming study.

Current Studies and Clinical Trials on Replacement Therapy for Beta Cells:

Objective: Promote the regeneration of existing beta cells or replace damaged beta cells in order to restore the body's capacity to make insulin.

Developments: Ongoing clinical studies investigating beta cells produced from stem cells and islet cells encapsulated to fend against immunological assault.

Gene Therapy:
The objective is to alter genes in order to improve the body's blood sugar regulation capabilities or

address the underlying causes of diabetes.

Progress: Preliminary human trials and animal models demonstrate the promise of this early study.

Intelligent Insulin:
The idea is to create insulin that reacts to blood sugar levels automatically. Preclinical and early clinical stages of experimental

formulations and delivery techniques represent progress.

The Prospects for Customised Medicine in the Treatment of Diabetes:
Method: Customising diabetes care according to each patient's unique genetic, environmental, and lifestyle characteristics.

Impact: Better treatment results by means of personalized drug schedules and lifestyle advice.

Non-invasive Monitoring of Blood Sugar:

Objective: Create gadgets that track blood sugar levels without requiring intrusive sensors or blood samples.

Research on sweat analysis, optical sensors, and other non-invasive technologies is progressing.

Both machine learning and artificial intelligence (AI):

Application: Make use of AI algorithms to evaluate massive datasets, forecast blood sugar patterns, enhance treatment regimens, and offer tailored advice.

Impact: More precision in insulin dosage, glucose monitoring, and general diabetes care.

CONCLUSION

Diabetes presents unique challenges, but with the right support network in place, it is possible to thrive and have a fulfilling life.

This conclusion emphasises the value of self-care, building a support network, being informed, and celebrating small victories in managing diabetes.

Effectively Managing Your Diabetes

Diabetes care requires dedication, perseverance, and adaptability and is a lifelong effort. Individuals with diabetes who monitor their blood sugar levels, follow medical advice, and adopt good lifestyle habits can lead active, fulfilling lives.

Crucial Advice for Effective Diabetes Management:

Healthy Eating: Consume a diet rich in fruits, vegetables, whole grains, and other nutrients that is well-balanced.

Regular Exercise: Engage in regular exercise to enhance blood sugar control, boost vitality, and enhance overall health.

Taking prescription
medications as directed and being open and honest with medical experts about any concerns or problems you may be experiencing are essential components of medication management.

Stress management:
Include stress-reduction techniques like mindfulness, meditation, and hobbies to

maintain emotional well-being.

Self-Monitoring: Pay careful attention to your blood sugar levels and log your development to identify patterns and adjust your treatment plan as necessary.

Establishing a Support Network

Having support from friends, family, and medical experts can help with diabetes management. Establishing a strong support network provides guidance, understanding, and encouragement.

How to Create a Support Network:

Educate Loved Ones:
Give your friends and family information on diabetes so they can help you manage the condition.

Engage in Support Groups:
 Use social media, online forums, or local support groups to connect with other people living with diabetes.

Seek Professional Assistance: Speak with healthcare providers who specialize in treating diabetes and who can offer tailored guidance and support.

Sustaining Education and Knowledge Knowing is powerful when it comes to treating diabetes. People may take control of their health and make informed decisions if they stay up to date on the latest research, treatments, and self-care practices.

Methods for Preserving Information:
Continuous Education
Learn as much as you can about diabetes from reputable sources, such as books, online resources, and medical journals.

Ask questions: Never hesitate to query medical professionals about your condition, potential therapies, and suggested lifestyle modifications.

Participate in workshops and seminars: Participate in training sessions, seminars, and webinars to increase your understanding of diabetes management.

Recognizing Successors and Important Occasions Diabetes management is an ongoing process with many highs and lows. No matter how small the victory, acknowledging it can motivate you and offer support as you proceed.

How to Give Acknowledgment for Success:

Create a strategy:
Establish reasonable goals and use benchmarks to track your progress.

Recognize Your Progress:
Take note of improvements in blood sugar control, general wellbeing, and lifestyle choices.

Reward Yourself:
Incentivize yourself with a special treat to

acknowledge reaching
milestones and overcoming
challenges.

APPENDICES

Living with diabetes presents unique challenges, but with the right approach and support, it's possible to thrive and maintain a fulfilling life. This conclusion highlights the importance of self-care, building a support network, staying informed, and celebrating successes in managing diabetes.

Living Well with Diabetes

Managing diabetes is a lifelong journey that requires dedication, resilience, and adaptability.

By adopting healthy lifestyle habits, monitoring blood sugar levels, and following medical advice, individuals with diabetes can lead active and fulfilling lives.

Key Strategies for Living Well with Diabetes:

Healthy Eating: Embrace a balanced diet rich in fruits, vegetables, lean proteins, and whole grains.

Regular Physical Activity: Engage in regular exercise to improve blood sugar control, boost energy levels, and enhance overall health.

Medication Management:
Take prescribed
medications as directed and
communicate openly with
healthcare providers about
any concerns or challenges.

Stress Management:
Incorporate stress-reduction
techniques such as
mindfulness, meditation,
and hobbies to maintain
emotional well-being.

Self-Monitoring:
Monitor blood sugar levels regularly and track progress to identify patterns and make informed adjustments to treatment plans.

Building a Support Network

Navigating diabetes management can be easier with the support of friends, family, and healthcare professionals. Building a

strong support network
provides encouragement,
guidance, and
understanding.

**Ways to Build a Support
Network:**
Educate Loved Ones: Help
friends and family
understand diabetes and
how they can support you in
managing the condition.

Join Support Groups:
Connect with others living with diabetes through local support groups, online forums, or social media communities.

Seek Professional Support:
Work with healthcare providers who specialize in diabetes care and can offer personalized guidance and support.

Staying Informed and Educated

Knowledge is empowering when it comes to managing diabetes. Staying informed about the latest research, treatment options, and self-care strategies can help individuals make informed decisions and advocate for their health.

Strategies for Staying Informed:

Continuous Learning: Stay updated on diabetes-related topics through reputable sources such as medical journals, books, and online resources.

Ask Questions: Don't hesitate to ask healthcare providers questions about your condition, treatment options, and lifestyle recommendations.

Attend Workshops and Seminars:
Participate in educational workshops, seminars, and webinars to deepen your understanding of diabetes management.

Celebrating Successes and Milestones

Managing diabetes is an ongoing journey filled with both challenges and achievements. Celebrating successes, no matter how small, can provide motivation and reinforcement along the way.

Ways to Celebrate Successes:

Set Goals: Establish achievable goals and celebrate milestones as you progress toward them.

Acknowledge Progress: Recognize improvements in blood sugar control, lifestyle habits, and overall well-being.

Reward Yourself:
Treat yourself to something special as a reward for reaching milestones and overcoming challenges.